Daily Fitness and Nutrition Journal

Boston   Burr Ridge, IL   Dubuque, IA   Madison, WI   New York
San Francisco   St. Louis   Bangkok   Bogotá   Caracas   Kuala Lumpur
Lisbon   London   Madrid   Mexico City   Milan   Montreal   New Delhi
Santiago   Seoul   Singapore   Sydney   Taipei   Toronto

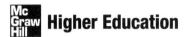

Higher Education

Daily Fitness and Nutrition Journal

1 2 3 4 5 6 7 8 9 0 FGR/FGR 0 9 8 7 6

ISBN-13: 978-0-07-302988-7
ISBN-10: 0-07-302988-2

www.mhhe.com

CONTENTS

FITNESS

Physical activity and exercise are key components of a wellness lifestyle. To live a long and healthy life, you must be active. The first part of this journal will help you develop a personalized plan for your fitness program. Once you are ready to put your plan into action, use the logs for weight training and for an overall exercise program to monitor the progress of your behavior change program.

First Steps

Before you begin to plan your fitness program, you should make sure that exercise is safe for you. If you are male and under 40 or female and under 50 and in good health, exercise is probably safe for you. If you are over these ages or have health problems, see your physician before starting an exercise program.

In addition, make sure that you are ready and motivated to increase your level of activity. Below, list the benefits and costs (pros and cons) of becoming more active and beginning a fitness program; include both short-term and long-term effects. Study your lists carefully. If you don't feel that the benefits of activity outweigh the costs, you'll have a more difficult time sticking with your program.

Benefits of increased physical activity:

_____

_____

_____

_____

_____

Costs of increased physical activity:

_____

_____

_____

_____

_____

Program Plans

1. *Determine your current fitness status and activity level.* Below, briefly describe your current fitness status and activity level. What types of physical activity do you currently engage in? At what intensity and for how long? If you've performed formal fitness testing as part of a wellness or health course, include a summary of the results below.

   Description of current activity/exercise habits:

   _____
   _____
   _____
   _____
   _____
   _____
   _____

   Results of fitness tests (test name and results):

   _____
   _____
   _____
   _____
   _____
   _____

   Are you satisfied with your current activity and fitness levels? Why or why not?

   _____
   _____
   _____
   _____
   _____
   _____
   _____

2. *Set goals.* Based on your analysis of the costs and benefits of fitness and your current activity and fitness levels, set goals for your fitness program. Your goals can be specific or general, short or long term. In the first section, include specific, measurable goals that you can use to track the progress of your fitness program. These goals might be things like raising your cardiorespiratory fitness rating, increasing daily steps (as measured with a pedometer), or swimming laps for 30 minutes without resting. In the second section, include long-term and more qualitative goals, such as improving the fit of your clothes and reducing your risk for chronic disease.

For each of your specific fitness goals, include a reward for achieving the goal. Rewards should be special, inexpensive, and preferably unrelated to food or alcohol.

Specific fitness goals:

1. Current status: _____ Goal: _____
   Target date: _____ Reward: _____
2. Current status: _____ Goal: _____
   Target date: _____ Reward: _____
3. Current status: _____ Goal: _____
   Target date: _____ Reward: _____
4. Current status: _____ Goal: _____
   Target date: _____ Reward: _____
5. Current status: _____ Goal: _____
   Target date: _____ Reward: _____

General goals:

1. _____
2. _____
3. _____
4. _____
5. _____

3. *Select activities.* Your program should be based around cardiorespiratory endurance exercise, but it should include activities that will develop all the different components of fitness. For example, your program might include bicycling, weight training, and stretching. Fill in the activities you've chosen on the overall program plan on the next page and check the components that each activity will develop.

   For weight training and stretching programs, you will need to select specific exercises to strengthen and stretch the different muscles of the body. Turn the page and fill in the exercises you've chosen for the weight training and stretching program plans. For each exercise in your weight training program, select a starting weight and number of repetitions and sets; add these to the "Weight Training Program Plan."

4. *Apply the FIT principle by setting a target frequency, intensity, and time for each activity.* Add these to the program plan on the next page. For advice on choosing activities and for determining appropriate frequency, intensity, and time (duration), refer to your textbook, visit the Web site of the American College of Sports Medicine (www.acsm.org), or consult an appropriate fitness professional.

5. *Begin and monitor your program.* Use the logs provided here to monitor your progress (see the weight training logs on pp. 8–23 and the overall fitness program logs on pp. 24–48). Be sure to complete the built-in progress check-ups every 6 weeks. To further track changes in your fitness status, record your starting resting heart rate (taken after 10 minutes of complete rest) in beats per minute and your blood pressure.

   Date: _____

   Resting heart rate: _____ bpm   Blood pressure: ____/____

Overall Program Plan

Activities	Components (Check ✔)					Frequency (Check ✔)							Intensity*	Time (Duration)
	Cardiorespiratory Endurance	Muscular Strength	Muscular Endurance	Flexibility	Body Composition	Monday	Tuesday	Wednesday	Thursday	Friday	Saturday	Sunday		
1.														
2.														
3.														
4.														
5.														
6.														

*You should conduct activities for achieving CRE goals in your target range for heart rate or RPE.

5

Weight Training Program Plan

Exercise	Muscle(s) developed	Weight (lb)	Repetitions	Sets

Stretching Program Plan

Exercise	Area(s) stretched

Weight Training Logs

Exercise/Date									
	Wt								
	Sets								
	Reps								
	Wt								
	Sets								
	Reps								
	Wt								
	Sets								
	Reps								
	Wt								
	Sets								
	Reps								
	Wt								
	Sets								
	Reps								
	Wt								
	Sets								
	Reps								
	Wt								
	Sets								
	Reps								
	Wt								
	Sets								
	Reps								
	Wt								
	Sets								
	Reps								
	Wt								
	Sets								
	Reps								
	Wt								
	Sets								
	Reps								
	Wt								
	Sets								
	Reps								

Wt												
Sets												
Reps												
Wt												
Sets												
Reps												
Wt												
Sets												
Reps												
Wt												
Sets												
Reps												
Wt												
Sets												
Reps												
Wt												
Sets												
Reps												
Wt												
Sets												
Reps												
Wt												
Sets												
Reps												
Wt												
Sets												
Reps												
Wt												
Sets												
Reps												
Wt												
Sets												
Reps												
Wt												
Sets												
Reps												

Exercise/Date								
	Wt							
	Sets							
	Reps							
	Wt							
	Sets							
	Reps							
	Wt							
	Sets							
	Reps							
	Wt							
	Sets							
	Reps							
	Wt							
	Sets							
	Reps							
	Wt							
	Sets							
	Reps							
	Wt							
	Sets							
	Reps							
	Wt							
	Sets							
	Reps							
	Wt							
	Sets							
	Reps							
	Wt							
	Sets							
	Reps							
	Wt							
	Sets							
	Reps							
	Wt							
	Sets							
	Reps							

Wt												
Sets												
Reps												
Wt												
Sets												
Reps												
Wt												
Sets												
Reps												
Wt												
Sets												
Reps												
Wt												
Sets												
Reps												
Wt												
Sets												
Reps												
Wt												
Sets												
Reps												
Wt												
Sets												
Reps												
Wt												
Sets												
Reps												
Wt												
Sets												
Reps												
Wt												
Sets												
Reps												

Exercise/Date									
	Wt								
	Sets								
	Reps								
	Wt								
	Sets								
	Reps								
	Wt								
	Sets								
	Reps								
	Wt								
	Sets								
	Reps								
	Wt								
	Sets								
	Reps								
	Wt								
	Sets								
	Reps								
	Wt								
	Sets								
	Reps								
	Wt								
	Sets								
	Reps								
	Wt								
	Sets								
	Reps								
	Wt								
	Sets								
	Reps								
	Wt								
	Sets								
	Reps								
	Wt								
	Sets								
	Reps								

Wt													
Sets														
Reps														
Wt														
Sets														
Reps														
Wt														
Sets														
Reps														
Wt														
Sets														
Reps														
Wt														
Sets														
Reps														
Wt														
Sets														
Reps														
Wt														
Sets														
Reps														
Wt														
Sets														
Reps														
Wt														
Sets														
Reps														
Wt														
Sets														
Reps														
Wt														
Sets														
Reps														

Exercise/Date									
	Wt								
	Sets								
	Reps								
	Wt								
	Sets								
	Reps								
	Wt								
	Sets								
	Reps								
	Wt								
	Sets								
	Reps								
	Wt								
	Sets								
	Reps								
	Wt								
	Sets								
	Reps								
	Wt								
	Sets								
	Reps								
	Wt								
	Sets								
	Reps								
	Wt								
	Sets								
	Reps								
	Wt								
	Sets								
	Reps								
	Wt								
	Sets								
	Reps								
	Wt								
	Sets								
	Reps								

Wt											
Sets											
Reps											
Wt											
Sets											
Reps											
Wt											
Sets											
Reps											
Wt											
Sets											
Reps											
Wt											
Sets											
Reps											
Wt											
Sets											
Reps											
Wt											
Sets											
Reps											
Wt											
Sets											
Reps											
Wt											
Sets											
Reps											
Wt											
Sets											
Reps											
Wt											
Sets											
Reps											
Wt											
Sets											
Reps											

Weight Training

Exercise/Date									
	Wt								
	Sets								
	Reps								
	Wt								
	Sets								
	Reps								
	Wt								
	Sets								
	Reps								
	Wt								
	Sets								
	Reps								
	Wt								
	Sets								
	Reps								
	Wt								
	Sets								
	Reps								
	Wt								
	Sets								
	Reps								
	Wt								
	Sets								
	Reps								
	Wt								
	Sets								
	Reps								
	Wt								
	Sets								
	Reps								
	Wt								
	Sets								
	Reps								
	Wt								
	Sets								
	Reps								

Wt												
Sets												
Reps												
Wt												
Sets												
Reps												
Wt												
Sets												
Reps												
Wt												
Sets												
Reps												
Wt												
Sets												
Reps												
Wt												
Sets												
Reps												
Wt												
Sets												
Reps												
Wt												
Sets												
Reps												
Wt												
Sets												
Reps												
Wt												
Sets												
Reps												
Wt												
Sets												
Reps												
Wt												
Sets												
Reps												

Exercise/Date									
	Wt								
	Sets								
	Reps								
	Wt								
	Sets								
	Reps								
	Wt								
	Sets								
	Reps								
	Wt								
	Sets								
	Reps								
	Wt								
	Sets								
	Reps								
	Wt								
	Sets								
	Reps								
	Wt								
	Sets								
	Reps								
	Wt								
	Sets								
	Reps								
	Wt								
	Sets								
	Reps								
	Wt								
	Sets								
	Reps								
	Wt								
	Sets								
	Reps								
	Wt								
	Sets								
	Reps								

Wt											
Sets											
Reps											
Wt											
Sets											
Reps											
Wt											
Sets											
Reps											
Wt											
Sets											
Reps											
Wt											
Sets											
Reps											
Wt											
Sets											
Reps											
Wt											
Sets											
Reps											
Wt											
Sets											
Reps											
Wt											
Sets											
Reps											
Wt											
Sets											
Reps											
Wt											
Sets											
Reps											
Wt											
Sets											
Reps											
Wt											
Sets											
Reps											

Exercise/Date									
	Wt								
	Sets								
	Reps								
	Wt								
	Sets								
	Reps								
	Wt								
	Sets								
	Reps								
	Wt								
	Sets								
	Reps								
	Wt								
	Sets								
	Reps								
	Wt								
	Sets								
	Reps								
	Wt								
	Sets								
	Reps								
	Wt								
	Sets								
	Reps								
	Wt								
	Sets								
	Reps								
	Wt								
	Sets								
	Reps								
	Wt								
	Sets								
	Reps								
	Wt								
	Sets								
	Reps								

Wt												
Sets												
Reps												
Wt												
Sets												
Reps												
Wt												
Sets												
Reps												
Wt												
Sets												
Reps												
Wt												
Sets												
Reps												
Wt												
Sets												
Reps												
Wt												
Sets												
Reps												
Wt												
Sets												
Reps												
Wt												
Sets												
Reps												
Wt												
Sets												
Reps												
Wt												
Sets												
Reps												

Exercise/Date									
	Wt								
	Sets								
	Reps								
	Wt								
	Sets								
	Reps								
	Wt								
	Sets								
	Reps								
	Wt								
	Sets								
	Reps								
	Wt								
	Sets								
	Reps								
	Wt								
	Sets								
	Reps								
	Wt								
	Sets								
	Reps								
	Wt								
	Sets								
	Reps								
	Wt								
	Sets								
	Reps								
	Wt								
	Sets								
	Reps								
	Wt								
	Sets								
	Reps								
	Wt								
	Sets								
	Reps								

Wt												
Sets												
Reps												
Wt												
Sets												
Reps												
Wt												
Sets												
Reps												
Wt												
Sets												
Reps												
Wt												
Sets												
Reps												
Wt												
Sets												
Reps												
Wt												
Sets												
Reps												
Wt												
Sets												
Reps												
Wt												
Sets												
Reps												
Wt												
Sets												
Reps												
Wt												
Sets												
Reps												
Wt												
Sets												
Reps												

Overall Fitness Program Logs

To use the overall fitness program logs, fill in the activities that are part of your program. Each day, note the distance and/or time you complete for each activity. For flexibility or weight training workouts, you may prefer just to enter a check mark each time you complete a workout. At the end of each week, total your distances and/or times. If you are tracking physical activity by counting steps with a pedometer, you can record daily steps and then calculate your weekly total or daily average steps.

SAMPLE

Date _____ Oct 18-24 _____

Activity	M	Tu	W	Th	F	Sa	Su	Weekly Total
1. Walking (time)	30	40	30	45				145 min
2. Weight training	✔		✔		✔			3 days
3. Stretching		✔		✔		✔		3 days
4. Swimming (yards)						800		800 yards
5.								
6.								

Fitness Program

24

Date _____

Activity	M	Tu	W	Th	F	Sa	Su	Weekly Total
1.								
2.								
3.								
4.								
5.								
6.								

Date _____

Activity	M	Tu	W	Th	F	Sa	Su	Weekly Total
1.								
2.								
3.								
4.								
5.								
6.								

Date _____

Activity	M	Tu	W	Th	F	Sa	Su	Weekly Total
1.								
2.								
3.								
4.								
5.								
6.								

Date _____

Activity	M	Tu	W	Th	F	Sa	Su	Weekly Total
1.								
2.								
3.								
4.								
5.								
6.								

Date _____

Activity	M	Tu	W	Th	F	Sa	Su	Weekly Total
1.								
2.								
3.								
4.								
5.								
6.								

Date _____

Activity	M	Tu	W	Th	F	Sa	Su	Weekly Total
1.								
2.								
3.								
4.								
5.								
6.								

Progress Check-Up: Week 6 of Program

Goals: Original Status   Current Status

_____   _____

_____   _____

_____   _____

_____   _____

_____   _____

Resting heart rate: _____ bpm   Blood pressure: ___/___

Below, list the activities in your program, and describe how satisfied you are with each activity and with your overall progress. List any problems you've encountered or any unexpected costs or benefits of your fitness program so far.

Activity: _____   Status: _____

_____

Activity: _____   Status: _____

_____

Activity: _____   Status: _____

_____

Activity: _____   Status: _____

_____

What is your overall response to your program so far? How do you feel about your program and its effects?

Fitness Program

Date _____

Activity	M	Tu	W	Th	F	Sa	Su	Weekly Total
1.								
2.								
3.								
4.								
5.								
6.								

Date _____

Activity	M	Tu	W	Th	F	Sa	Su	Weekly Total
1.								
2.								
3.								
4.								
5.								
6.								

Date _____

Activity	M	Tu	W	Th	F	Sa	Su	Weekly Total
1.								
2.								
3.								
4.								
5.								
6.								

Date _____

Activity	M	Tu	W	Th	F	Sa	Su	Weekly Total
1.								
2.								
3.								
4.								
5.								
6.								

Date _____

Activity	M	Tu	W	Th	F	Sa	Su	Weekly Total
1.								
2.								
3.								
4.								
5.								
6.								

Date _____

Activity	M	Tu	W	Th	F	Sa	Su	Weekly Total
1.								
2.								
3.								
4.								
5.								
6.								

Progress Check-Up: Week 12 of Program

Goals: Original Status   Current Status

_____	_____
_____	_____
_____	_____
_____	_____

Resting heart rate: _____ bpm   Blood pressure: ____/____

Below, list the activities in your program, and describe how satisfied you are with each activity and with your overall progress. List any problems you've encountered or any unexpected costs or benefits of your fitness program so far.

Activity: _____   Status: _____

Activity: _____   Status: _____

Activity: _____   Status: _____

Activity: _____   Status: _____

What is your overall response to your program so far? How do you feel about your program and its effects?

Fitness Program

Date _____

Activity	M	Tu	W	Th	F	Sa	Su	Weekly Total
1.								
2.								
3.								
4.								
5.								
6.								

Date _____

Activity	M	Tu	W	Th	F	Sa	Su	Weekly Total
1.								
2.								
3.								
4.								
5.								
6.								

Date _____

Activity	M	Tu	W	Th	F	Sa	Su	Weekly Total
1.								
2.								
3.								
4.								
5.								
6.								

Date _____

Activity	M	Tu	W	Th	F	Sa	Su	Weekly Total
1.								
2.								
3.								
4.								
5.								
6.								

Date _____

Activity	M	Tu	W	Th	F	Sa	Su	Weekly Total
1.								
2.								
3.								
4.								
5.								
6.								

Date _____

Activity	M	Tu	W	Th	F	Sa	Su	Weekly Total
1.								
2.								
3.								
4.								
5.								
6.								

Progress Check-Up: Week 18 of Program

Goals: Original Status   Current Status

_____   _____

_____   _____

_____   _____

_____   _____

_____   _____

Resting heart rate: _____ bpm Blood pressure: ____/____

Below, list the activities in your program, and describe how satisfied you are with each activity and with your overall progress. List any problems you've encountered or any unexpected costs or benefits of your fitness program so far.

Activity: _____   Status: _____

_____

Activity: _____   Status: _____

_____

Activity: _____   Status: _____

_____

Activity: _____   Status: _____

_____

What is your overall response to your program so far? How do you feel about your program and its effects?

Date _____

Activity	M	Tu	W	Th	F	Sa	Su	Weekly Total
1.								
2.								
3.								
4.								
5.								
6.								

Date _____

Activity	M	Tu	W	Th	F	Sa	Su	Weekly Total
1.								
2.								
3.								
4.								
5.								
6.								

Date _____

Activity	M	Tu	W	Th	F	Sa	Su	Weekly Total
1.								
2.								
3.								
4.								
5.								
6.								

Date _____

Activity	M	Tu	W	Th	F	Sa	Su	Weekly Total
1.								
2.								
3.								
4.								
5.								
6.								

Date _____

Activity	M	Tu	W	Th	F	Sa	Su	Weekly Total
1.								
2.								
3.								
4.								
5.								
6.								

Fitness Program

Date _____

Activity	M	Tu	W	Th	F	Sa	Su	Weekly Total
1.								
2.								
3.								
4.								
5.								
6.								

Progress Check-Up: Week 24 of Program

Goals: Original Status   Current Status

_____   _____

_____   _____

_____   _____

_____   _____

_____   _____

Resting heart rate: _____ bpm   Blood pressure: ____/____

Below, list the activities in your program, and describe how satisfied you are with each activity and with your overall progress. List any problems you've encountered or any unexpected costs or benefits of your fitness program so far.

Activity: _____   Status: _____

_____

Activity: _____   Status: _____

_____

Activity: _____   Status: _____

_____

Activity: _____   Status: _____

_____

What is your overall response to your program so far? How do you feel about your program and its effects?

Date _____

Activity	M	Tu	W	Th	F	Sa	Su	Weekly Total
1.								
2.								
3.								
4.								
5.								
6.								

Date _____

Activity	M	Tu	W	Th	F	Sa	Su	Weekly Total
1.								
2.								
3.								
4.								
5.								
6.								

Date _____

Activity	M	Tu	W	Th	F	Sa	Su	Weekly Total
1.								
2.								
3.								
4.								
5.								
6.								

Date _____

Activity	M	Tu	W	Th	F	Sa	Su	Weekly Total
1.								
2.								
3.								
4.								
5.								
6.								

Date _____

Activity	M	Tu	W	Th	F	Sa	Su	Weekly Total
1.								
2.								
3.								
4.								
5.								
6.								

Date _____

Activity	M	Tu	W	Th	F	Sa	Su	Weekly Total
1.								
2.								
3.								
4.								
5.								
6.								

Progress Check-Up: Week 30 of Program

Goals: Original Status   Current Status

_____   _____

_____   _____

_____   _____

_____   _____

_____   _____

Resting heart rate: _____ bpm Blood pressure: ____/____

Below, list the activities in your program, and describe how satisfied you are with each activity and with your overall progress. List any problems you've encountered or any unexpected costs or benefits of your fitness program so far.

Activity: _____ Status: _____
_____

Activity: _____ Status: _____
_____

Activity: _____ Status: _____
_____

Activity: _____ Status: _____
_____

What is your overall response to your program so far? How do you feel about your program and its effects?

Date _____

Activity	M	Tu	W	Th	F	Sa	Su	Weekly Total
1.								
2.								
3.								
4.								
5.								
6.								

Date _____

Activity	M	Tu	W	Th	F	Sa	Su	Weekly Total
1.								
2.								
3.								
4.								
5.								
6.								

Date _____

Activity	M	Tu	W	Th	F	Sa	Su	Weekly Total
1.								
2.								
3.								
4.								
5.								
6.								

Date _____

Activity	M	Tu	W	Th	F	Sa	Su	Weekly Total
1.								
2.								
3.								
4.								
5.								
6.								

Date _____

Activity	M	Tu	W	Th	F	Sa	Su	Weekly Total
1.								
2.								
3.								
4.								
5.								
6.								

Date _____

Activity	M	Tu	W	Th	F	Sa	Su	Weekly Total
1.								
2.								
3.								
4.								
5.								
6.								

Progress Check-Up: Week 36 of Program

Goals: Original Status   Current Status

_____   _____

_____   _____

_____   _____

_____   _____

_____   _____

Resting heart rate: _____ bpm Blood pressure: ____/____

Below, list the activities in your program, and describe how satisfied you are with each activity and with your overall progress. List any problems you've encountered or any unexpected costs or benefits of your fitness program so far.

Activity: _____ Status: _____

_____

Activity: _____ Status: _____

_____

Activity: _____ Status: _____

_____

Activity: _____ Status: _____

_____

What is your overall response to your program so far? How do you feel about your program and its effects? Do you think you will stick with your program? Why or why not?

NUTRITION

Nutrition is a vitally important component of wellness. Diet influences energy levels, well-being, and overall health. A well-planned diet supports maximum fitness and protects against disease. This part of your journal will help you analyze your current eating habits, identify patterns that may be causing you to shortchange yourself on nutrition, and put a more balanced eating plan into action.

To start monitoring, assessing, and improving your nutritional habits, follow these steps:

1. Review the tools for keeping a nutrition log provided on pages 50–60.
2. Using these tools, fill out the Preprogram Nutrition Log for 3 days.
3. Use the Assessing Your Daily Diet worksheets to analyze your daily nutritional intake. Do you see some areas in your current diet that could be improved?
4. Complete the Behavior Change Contract. The information in the Tools for Improving Your Food Choices section will help you identify unhealthy behaviors and plan how to improve them.
5. Record your daily diet a second time in the Postprogram Nutrition Log.
6. Analyze your revised diet and compare it to your original diet.

Once you understand your nutritional needs and habits, you can make reasonable and healthy choices for weight management. Additional nutrition log pages are provided for longer-term monitoring of your diet.

TOOLS FOR MONITORING YOUR DAILY DIET

MyPyramid Food Guidance System

The latest version of the USDA daily food guide, released in 2005, is called MyPyramid. The MyPyramid food guidance system can help you get the most nutrition out of your calories and make smart choices from every food group. It emphasizes that consuming a balance of servings from each group will both meet the body's nutritional needs and help reduce chronic disease risk. The MyPyramid symbol is shown below, along with the recommended food group intakes for a 2000-calorie diet; for information on specific, personalized recommendations, refer to the following page.

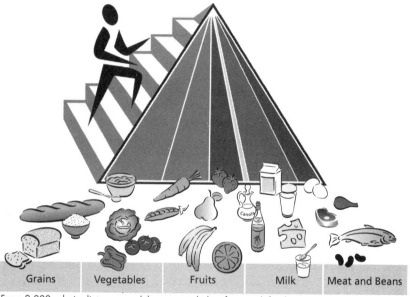

Grains	Vegetables	Fruits	Milk	Meat and Beans

For a 2,000-calorie diet, you need the amounts below from each food group. To find the amounts that are right for you, go to MyPyramid.gov.

Eat 6 oz. very day	Eat 2½ cups every day	Eat 2 cups every day	Get 3 cups every day for kids aged 2 to 8, it's 2	Eat 5½ oz. every day

Figure 1 MyPyramid

SOURCE: U.S. Department of Agriculture. 2005. MyPyramid (http://mypyramid.gov; retrieved April 20, 2005).

Nutrition

Recommended MyPyramid Food Group Intakes

The number of servings you should consume from each group depends on your overall calorie intake and activity level. For example, an active 18-year-old male would need to consume more calories than a sedentary 60-year-old female for weight maintenance. For guidance in determining an appropriate calorie intake and food intake pattern for yourself, refer to your text and/or the MyPyramid.gov Web site. At the site, you can answer a few questions and receive a personalized recommendation.

Based on information from your text or the MyPyramid.gov site, fill in the right column in the chart of recommendations below:

Group	Recommended Daily Intake: Sample for 2000-Calorie Diet	Recommended Daily Intake: Your Calorie Level
Daily Energy Intake	2000 calories	____ calories
Grains	6 oz-eq	____ oz-eq
Whole grains	3 oz-eq	____ oz-eq
Other grains	3 oz-eq	____ oz-eq
Vegetables	2.5 cups	____ cups
Fruits	2 cups	____ cups
Milk	3 cups	____ cups
Meat and Beans	5.5 oz-eq	____ oz-eq
Oils	6 tsp	____ tsp
Discretionary Calories*	267 calories	____ calories
Solid fats	18 g	____ g
Added sugars	32 g (8 tsp)	____ g (____ tsp)

*The suggested intakes from the basic food groups in MyPyramid assume that nutrient-dense forms are selected from each group; nutrient-dense forms are those that are fat-free or low-fat and that contain no added sugars. If this pattern is followed, then a small amount of additional calories can be consumed—the discretionary calorie allowance. The allowance at your calorie intake level—and how it might divided between solid fats and added sugars—is listed in your text and on the MyPyramid.gov site.

Estimating Food Intake
MyPyramid Portion Sizes Guide

To compare your diet to that recommended for your calorie intake, you need to track your portion sizes according to consistent measures. Use the information in this chart to more accurately track your daily food intake.

Foods and Portion Size Measures	Serving Size Equivalents
Grains Group 1 oz equivalent = • 1 slice bread • 1 small muffin • 1 cup ready-to-eat cereal flakes • 1/2 cup cooked cereal, rice, or pasta • 1 6-inch tortilla	• 1/2 cup of rice = an ice cream scoop or one-third of a soda can • 1 cup pasta = a small adult fist or a tennis ball • 1/2 oz muffin or roll = a plum or large egg • 1 oz bagel = a hockey puck or yo-yo • 1 tortilla = diameter of a small plate
Vegetable Group 1/2 cup or equivalent (1 serving) = • 1/2 cup cooked or raw vegetables • 1 cup raw leafy vegetables • 1/2 cup tomato sauce • 1/2 cup vegetable juice	• 1/2 cup cooked vegetables = an ice cream scoop or one-third of a soda can • 1/2 cup juice = one-third of a soda can • 1 medium potato = computer mouse The following count as 1 cup: 3 broccoli spears, 1 large tomato, 1 ear of corn, 12 baby carrots, 2 large celery stalks, 1 medium potato

Fruit Group $^1/_2$ cup or equivalent (1 serving) = • $^1/_2$ cup fresh, canned, or frozen fruit • $^1/_2$ cup fruit juice • 1 small whole fruit • $^1/_4$ cup dried fruit	• 1 medium fruit = a baseball • $^1/_2$ cup fruit = an ice cream scoop or one-third of a soda can • $^1/_2$ cup juice = one-third of a soda can The following count as 1 cup: 1 large banana, 8 strawberries, 32 grapes, 12 melon balls, $^1/_4$ medium cantaloupe
Milk Group 1 cup or equivalent = • 1 cup milk or yogurt • $1^1/_2$ oz natural cheese • 2 oz processed cheese	• 1 oz cheese = your thumb, 4 dice, or an ice cube
Meat and Beans Group 1 oz equivalent = • 1 oz cooked lean meat, poultry, or fish • $^1/_4$ cup cooked dry beans or tofu • 1 egg • 1 tablespoon peanut butter • $^1/_2$ oz nuts or seeds	• 3 oz chicken or meat = deck of cards or an audiocassette tape • $^1/_2$ cup cooked beans = an ice cream scoop or one-third of a soda can • 2 tablespoons peanut butter = a Ping-Pong ball or large marshmallow • $^1/_4$ cup seeds = golf ball
Oils 1 teaspoon or equivalent = • 1 teaspoon vegetable oil • 1 tablespoon salad dressing or light mayonnaise	• 1 teaspoon margarine = tip of thumb The following food portions contain about 1 teaspoon of oil: 8 large olives, $^1/_6$ medium avocado, $^1/_2$ tablespoon peanut butter, $^1/_3$ ounce roasted nuts

Additional guidelines for estimating food intake and counting discretionary calories are available at MyPyramid.gov.

Making Choices Within the Food Groups

The average American diet is at or below the recommended intake from most food groups, but we eat too much fat and added sugars to meet the recommendations without gaining weight. The key is to make better food choices within the groups and so get more nutrients for your calories. Keep these guidelines in mind as you plan your meals:

General

- Choose a variety of foods within each group. Different foods contain different combinations of nutrients.
- If you are concerned about eating too much and gaining weight, concentrate on nutrient-dense foods— foods that are high in nutrients relative to the amount of calories they contain.

Grains: Make Half Your Grains Whole

Americans currently consume an average of about 1 serving of whole grains per day. MyPyramid recommends that half of all grain servings be whole grains, a minimum of 3 servings of whole-grain foods per day. Whole grains include the following:

- whole wheat
- whole rye
- whole oats
- oatmeal
- whole-grain corn
- popcorn
- brown rice
- whole-grain barley
- bulgur (cracked wheat)
- millet
- kasha
- quinoa
- wheat and rye berries
- amaranth
- wild rice
- whole-grain spelt and kamut

Wheat flour, unbleached flour, enriched flour, and degerminated corn meal are not whole grains.

Additional tips for this group:

- Choose foods that contain little fat or sugar, such as bread, rice, or pasta.

- Limit foods that are high in fat and sugar such as pastries, croissants, cakes, and cookies.

Vegetables: Vary Your Veggies

Because vegetables vary in the nutrients they provide, it is important to consume a variety of types of vegetables to obtain maximum nutrition. To help boost variety, MyPyramid recommends servings from five different subgroups within the vegetables group; try to consume vegetables from several subgroups each day:

- Dark green vegetables like spinach, chard, collards, bok choy, broccoli, kale, romaine, chicory, endive, and turnip, beet, dandelion, and mustard greens
- Orange and deep yellow vegetables like carrots, winter squash, sweet potatoes, and pumpkin
- Legumes like pinto beans, kidney beans, black beans, navy beans, black-eyed peas, lentils, chickpeas, soybeans, split peas, and tofu (legumes can be counted as servings of vegetables or as alternatives to meat)
- Starchy vegetables like corn, green peas, hominy, lima beans, taro, and white potatoes
- Other vegetables; tomatoes, bell peppers (red, orange, yellow, or green), green beans, and cruciferous vegetables like cauliflower are good choices

In addition to choosing a variety of vegetables, limit the fat you add to vegetables during cooking and at the table as spreads and toppings.

Fruits: Focus on Fruits

- Choose whole fruits more often than juices; choose fruit juices over fruit punches, ades, and drinks.
- For canned fruits, choose those packed in 100% fruit juice rather than in syrup.
- Citrus fruits, melons, bananas, and berries are particularly good choices.

Nutrition

Milk: Get Your Calcium-Rich Foods

This group includes all milk and milk products, such as yogurt, cheeses (except cream cheese), and dairy desserts, as well as lactose-free and lactose-reduced products.

- Choose servings of low-fat and fat-free items from this group. Limit serving sizes of high-fat choices.
- Cottage cheese is lower in calcium than most cheeses.
- For those who choose not to consume dairy products, calcium is also found in fortified breads and breakfast cereals, dried fruits, green leafy vegetables, legumes, and some soy foods.

Meat and Beans: Go Lean with Protein

This group includes meat, poultry, fish, dry beans and peas, eggs, nuts, and seeds.

- Choose lean cuts of meat and skinless poultry, and trim away all the fat you can see. Watch your serving sizes carefully.
- Choose at least one serving of plant proteins, such as black beans, lentils, or tofu, every day.

Oils

The oils group represents the oils that are added to foods during processing, cooking, or at the table; oils and soft margarines include vegetable oils and soft vegetable oil table spreads that have no trans fats. Foods that are mostly oils include nuts, olives, avocados, and some fish.

- Limit your intake of oils to the recommended MyPyramid amount for your level of calorie intake.
- Remember that solid (saturated) fats are counted as discretionary calories.

Discretionary Calories—Solid Fats and Added Sugars

The suggested intakes from the basic food groups in MyPyramid assume that nutrient-dense forms—those that are fat-free or low-fat and that contain no added sugars—are selected

Nutrition

from each group. If this pattern is followed, then a small amount of additional calories can be consumed—the discretionary calorie allowance. People who are trying to lose weight may choose not to use discretionary calories.

For those wanting to maintain weight, discretionary calories may be used to increase the amount of food from a food group; to consume foods that are not in the lowest fat form or that contain added sugars; or to add oil, fat, or sugars to foods. Examples of discretionary solid fat calories include choosing higher-fat meats such as sausages or chicken with skin, choosing whole milk instead of fat-free milk, and topping foods with butter. Added sugars are found in sweetened beverages (regular soda, sweetened teas, fruit drinks), dairy products (ice cream, some yogurts), and grain products (bakery goods).

Additional Resources

There are many Web sites with advice for making healthy shopping and food choices, as well as many sites presenting basic cooking skills and recipes. The following are just a few online resources that can help you improve your diet:

American Heart Association
www.deliciousdecisions.org
Dietary Guidelines for Americans
www.healthierus.gov/nutrition.html
MyPyramid.gov
www.mypyramid.gov
National Cancer Institute: Eat 5 to 9 a Day
www.5aday.gov/recipes
National Heart, Lung, and Blood Institute (search for "recipes" and "Go, Slow, and Whoa" foods)
www.nhlbi.nih.gov
Student Nosh
www.studentnosh.com
U.S. Department of Agriculture
www.nutrition.gov
Yum Yum: Student Recipes
www.yumyum.com/student

Self-Assessment: Portion Size Quiz

Now test your perception of portion sizes (check your answers on the next page).

1. An ounce and a half of hard cheese—equivalent to one cup from the milk group—looks most like
   a. one domino.
   b. two dominoes.
   c. three dominoes.

2. A half cup of cooked pasta, considered an ounce-equivalent from the grain group, most easily fits into
   a. an ice cream scoop (the kind with a release handle).
   b. a ball the size of a medium grapefruit.
   c. a cereal bowl.

3. One drink of wine roughly fills
   a. two-thirds of a coffee cup.
   b. one coffee cup.
   c. two coffee cups.

4. One ½-cup serving of green grapes consists of how many grapes?
   a. 10
   b. 15
   c. 20

5. Three ounces of beef most closely resembles
   a. a *T.V. Guide.*
   b. a regular bar of soap.
   c. a small bar of soap (as from a hotel).

6. One ½-cup serving of brussels sprouts consists of how many sprouts?
   a. 4
   b. 8
   c. 12

7. Two tablespoons of olive oil more or less fill
   a. a shot glass.
   b. a thimble.
   c. a Dixie cup.

8. Two tablespoons of peanut butter make a ball the size of
   a. a marble.
   b. a tennis ball.
   c. a Ping-Pong ball.

9. How many shakes of a five-hole salt shaker does it take to reach 1 teaspoon (approximately the maximum amount of salt recommended per day)?
   a. 5
   b. 10
   c. 60

10. There are eight servings in a loaf of Entenmann's Raspberry Danish Twist. A serving is the width of
    a. one finger.
    b. two fingers.
    c. four fingers.

Answers

| 1. c | 3. a | 5. b | 7. a | 9. c |
| 2. a | 4. b | 6. a | 8. c | 10. b |

Source: What's in a Portion? *Tufts University Diet and Nutrition Letter,* September, 1994. Reprinted with permission, *Tufts University Health and Nutrition Letter* (1-800-274-7581).

Reading Food Labels

Another important tool for keeping your nutrition log is the information you will find on food labels. In the example on page 60, note that the serving size is 1 cup. If you eat 2 cups of chili, you'll need to double all the values on the label. Other useful information includes total calories and calories from fat per serving. Remember that the serving size given on the food label is often not the same as the size of the portion you choose for yourself.

Nutrition

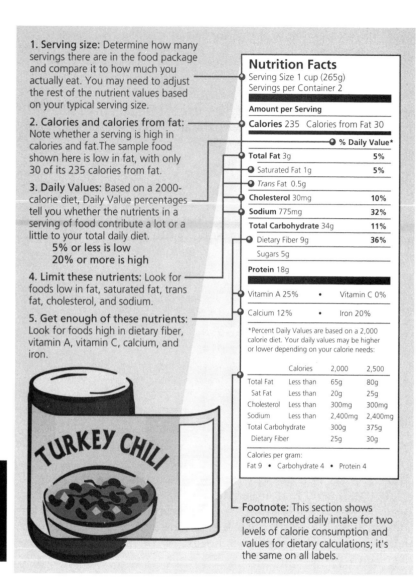

1. **Serving size:** Determine how many servings there are in the food package and compare it to how much you actually eat. You may need to adjust the rest of the nutrient values based on your typical serving size.

2. **Calories and calories from fat:** Note whether a serving is high in calories and fat. The sample food shown here is low in fat, with only 30 of its 235 calories from fat.

3. **Daily Values:** Based on a 2000-calorie diet, Daily Value percentages tell you whether the nutrients in a serving of food contribute a lot or a little to your total daily diet.
   5% or less is low
   20% or more is high

4. **Limit these nutrients:** Look for foods low in fat, saturated fat, trans fat, cholesterol, and sodium.

5. **Get enough of these nutrients:** Look for foods high in dietary fiber, vitamin A, vitamin C, calcium, and iron.

Footnote: This section shows recommended daily intake for two levels of calorie consumption and values for dietary calculations; it's the same on all labels.

Nutrition Facts

Serving Size 1 cup (265g)
Servings per Container 2

Amount per Serving

Calories 235   Calories from Fat 30

	% Daily Value*
Total Fat 3g	**5%**
Saturated Fat 1g	**5%**
Trans Fat 0.5g	
Cholesterol 30mg	**10%**
Sodium 775mg	**32%**
Total Carbohydrate 34g	**11%**
Dietary Fiber 9g	**36%**
Sugars 5g	
Protein 18g	

Vitamin A 25%	•	Vitamin C 0%
Calcium 12%	•	Iron 20%

*Percent Daily Values are based on a 2,000 calorie diet. Your daily values may be higher or lower depending on your calorie needs:

	Calories	2,000	2,500
Total Fat	Less than	65g	80g
Sat Fat	Less than	20g	25g
Cholesterol	Less than	300mg	300mg
Sodium	Less than	2,400mg	2,400mg
Total Carbohydrate		300g	375g
Dietary Fiber		25g	30g

Calories per gram:
Fat 9 • Carbohydrate 4 • Protein 4

Figure 2. Food Label

PREPROGRAM NUTRITION LOGS

Use the preprogram nutrition logs to keep track of everything you eat for 3 consecutive days. Break down each food item into its component parts and list them separately in the column labeled "Food." Then enter the portion size you consume in the correct food group column; refer to the chart on pages 52–53. For example, a turkey sandwich might be listed as follows: whole-wheat bread, 2 oz-equiv of whole grains; turkey, 2 oz-equiv of meat/beans; tomato, $\frac{1}{3}$ cup vegetables; romaine lettuce, $\frac{1}{4}$ cup vegetables; 1 tablespoon mayonnaise dressing, 1 teaspoon oils. It can be challenging to track values for added sugars and, especially, oils and fats, but use food labels and information in Appendixes B and C in your text to be as accurate as you can. MyPyramid.gov has additional guidelines for counting discretionary calories. At the bottom of the chart, keep count of the number of servings of whole grains and the number of vegetable subgroups you consume daily (whole grains and vegetable subgroups are described on pp. 54–55).

Nutrition

Preprogram Nutrition Log

DAY 1

Food	Grains (oz-eq)	Vegetables (cups)	Fruit (cups)	Milk (cups)	Meat/beans (oz-eq)	Oils (tsp)	Solid fats (g)	Added sugars (g/tsp)
Daily total								

Number of servings of whole grains: ____
Number of vegetable subgroups consumed: ____

Preprogram Nutrition Log

DAY 2

Food	Grains (oz-eq)	Vegetables (cups)	Fruit (cups)	Milk (cups)	Meat/beans (oz-eq)	Oils (tsp)	Solid fats (g)	Added sugars (g/tsp)
Daily total								

Number of servings of whole grains: ____
Number of vegetable subgroups consumed: ____

Preprogram Nutrition Log

DAY 3

Food	Grains (oz-eq)	Vegetables (cups)	Fruit (cups)	Milk (cups)	Meat/beans (oz-eq)	Oils (tsp)	Solid fats (g)	Added sugars (g/tsp)
Daily total								

Number of servings of whole grains: ____
Number of vegetable subgroups consumed: ____

ASSESSING YOUR DAILY DIET

A balanced diet follows the MyPyramid recommendations. Fill in your recommended MyPyramid intakes from p. 51 and then the daily totals from your 3 days of preprogram food logs. Average your daily totals and compare them to the MyPyramid recommendations.

Group	Day 1	Day 2	Day 3	Average of 3 Days	MyPyramid recommended totals
Grains (oz-eq)					
Whole grains (oz-eq)					
Vegetables (cups)					
# of subgroups					*
Fruit (cups)					
Milk (cups)					
Meat/beans (oz-eq)					
Oils (tsp)					
Solid fats (g)					
Added sugars (g/tsp)					

* To consume the recommended variety of vegetables, you should eat vegetables from several (3–5) subgroups each day; the five subgroups are described on p. 55.

How does your diet compare to the recommended intakes for your level of energy intake?

Nutrition

NUTRITION BEHAVIOR CHANGE CONTRACT

Have you identified some areas of your diet where you don't meet the MyPyramid recommendations? Perhaps you have more than the recommended amount of added sugars in your diet or don't eat enough vegetables. Take a good look at your current diet and think about the changes you can make to improve it. Use the Behavior Change Contract on the next page to record your plan for dietary change and the steps that you will follow to reach your goal.

1. Fill in your name and your target for change. Examples of behavior change targets include increasing daily servings of vegetables and decreasing intake of added sugars.

2. Enter a start date, final goal, and target completion date. Allow enough time to achieve your overall goal. Make your goal specific, such as increasing fruit intake from 2 servings per week to 3 servings per day.

3. Break your program into several stages and give yourself a reward for achieving each mini-goal in addition to a reward for reaching your final goal.

4. List specific strategies for achieving your goal, including such things as packing fruit in your backpack every morning, getting up 15 minutes earlier to allow time for a sit-down breakfast, and stocking your refrigerator with healthy beverages. Your program will probably involve making trade-offs: Review your nutrition logs and identify foods high in fat and sugar and low in other nutrients; these are foods to target for reduction or elimination. For additional tips, go to the Tools for Improving Your Food Choices section and use the quizzes and tables there (pp. 68–72).

5. Use the logs provided in this journal or develop your own plan for monitoring your eating habits and the progress of your program.

6. Sign your contract and, if possible, recruit a witness who can also participate in your program. (Your helper might eat a meal with you each day or call to offer encouragement.)

Behavior Change Contract

1. I _____ agree to
_____

2. I will begin on _____ and plan to reach my

goal of _____ by _____

3. In order to reach my final goal, I have devised the following schedule of mini-goals. For each step in my program, I will give myself the reward listed:

Mini-goal	Target date	Reward
_____	_____	_____
_____	_____	_____
_____	_____	_____

My overall reward for reaching my final goal will be
_____

4. My plan for reaching my goal includes the following strategies:
_____
_____
_____
_____
_____

5. I will use the following tools to monitor my progress toward reaching my final goal:
_____
_____

I sign this contract as an indication of my personal commitment to reach my goal.

Your signature: _____ Date: _____

I have recruited a helper who will witness my contract and
_____
_____

Witness signature: _____ Date: _____

TOOLS FOR IMPROVING YOUR FOOD CHOICES

Dietary Guidelines for Americans

As you plan to change your diet, keep in mind the Dietary Guidelines for Americans. These guidelines, which are described in more detail in your textbook and online (www.healthierus.gov/nutrition.html), provide a good foundation for a lifestyle that promotes health.

- Consume a variety of nutrient-dense foods within and among the basic food groups, while staying within energy needs.

- Control calorie intake to manage body weight.

- Be physically active every day.

- Increase daily intake of foods from certain groups: fruits and vegetables, whole grains, and fat-free or low-fat milk and milk products.

- Choose fats wisely for good health, limiting intake of saturated and trans fats.

- Choose carbohydrates wisely for good health, limiting intake of added sugars.

- Choose and prepare foods with little salt, and consume potassium-rich foods.

- If you drink alcoholic beverages, do so in moderation.

- Keep foods safe to eat.

Making Healthy Ethnic Food Choices

	Choose Often	**Choose Seldom**
Chinese	Chinese greens Hunan or Szechuan dishes Rice, brown or white Steamed dishes Stir-fry dishes Wonton soup	Crispy duck or beef Egg rolls or fried wontons General Tso's chicken Kung pao dishes Rice, fried Sweet-and-sour dishes
Italian	Cioppino (seafood stew) Minestrone soup, vegetarian Pasta with marinara sauce Pasta primavera Pasta with red or white clam sauce	Cannelloni, ravioli, or manicotti Fettucini alfredo Fried calamari Garlic bread Veal or eggplant parmigiana
Indian	Chapati (baked tortilla-like bread) Dal (lentils) Karhi (chick-pea soup) Khur (milk and rice dessert) Tandoori, chicken or fish Yogurt-based curry dishes	Bhatura, poori, or paratha (fried breads) Coconut milk-based dishes Ghee (clarified butter) Korma (rich meat dish) Pakoras (fried appetizer) Samosa (fried meat and vegetables in dough)
Japanese	Kushiyaki (broiled foods on skewers) Shabu-shabu (foods in boiling broth) Sushi	Agemono (deep-fried foods) Sukiyaki Tonkatsu (fried pork) Tempura (fried chicken, shrimp, or vegetables)

Nutrition

69

	Choose Often	**Choose Seldom**
Mexican	Beans and rice	Chiles relleños
	Black bean and	Chimichangas or
	vegetable soup	flautas
	Burritos, bean or	Enchiladas, beef or
	chicken	cheese
	Fajitas, chicken or	Nachos or fried
	vegetable	tortillas
	Gazpacho	Quesadillas
	Refried beans,	Refried beans made
	nonfat or low-fat	with lard
	Tortillas, steamed	Taco salad
Thai	Forest salad	Fried fish, duck, or
	Larb (chicken salad	chicken
	with mint)	Curries with coconut
	Po tak (seafood	milk
	stew)	Dishes with peanut
	Yum neua (broiled	sauce
	beef with onions)	Yum koon chaing
		(sausage with peppers)

Source: The sat fat switch; 1997. *Nutrition Action Healthletter,* January/February. University of Southern Florida University of Southern Florida Student Health Service. 1997. Ethnic food (http://www.shs/usf.edu/Health/ethnic.html). The best of Asian cuisines, 1993; *University of California at Berkeley Wellness Letter,* January. Eating in ethnic restaurants, 1990; *Runner's World,* January. Reprinted by permission of *Runner's World Magazine.*

Self-Assessment: What Triggers Your Eating?

Hunger isn't the only reason people eat. Efforts to make healthy eating choices can be sabotaged by eating related to other factors, such as emotions or patterns of thinking. Your score on this quiz will help you understand your motivations for eating so that you can create an effective plan for changing your eating behavior. Circle the number that indicates to what degree each situation is likely to make you start eating.

Nutrition

Social	Very Unlikely Very Likely
1. Arguing or being in conflict with someone	1 2 3 4 5 6 7 8 9 10
2. Being with others when they are eating	1 2 3 4 5 6 7 8 9 10
3. Being urged to eat by someone else	1 2 3 4 5 6 7 8 9 10

Social (continued)

	Very Unlikely						Very Likely			
4. Feeling inadequate around others	1	2	3	4	5	6	7	8	9	10

Emotional

5. Feeling bad, such as being anxious or depressed	1	2	3	4	5	6	7	8	9	10
6. Feeling good, happy, or relaxed	1	2	3	4	5	6	7	8	9	10
7. Feeling bored or having time on my hands	1	2	3	4	5	6	7	8	9	10
8. Feeling stressed or excited	1	2	3	4	5	6	7	8	9	10

Situational

9. Seeing an advertisement for food or eating	1	2	3	4	5	6	7	8	9	10
10. Passing by a bakery, cookie shop, or other enticement to eat	1	2	3	4	5	6	7	8	9	10
11. Being involved in a party, celebration, or special occasion	1	2	3	4	5	6	7	8	9	10
12. Eating out	1	2	3	4	5	6	7	8	9	10

Thinking

13. Making excuses to myself about why it's okay to eat	1	2	3	4	5	6	7	8	9	10
14. Berating myself for being so fat or unable to control my eating	1	2	3	4	5	6	7	8	9	10
15. Worrying about others or about difficulties I am having	1	2	3	4	5	6	7	8	9	10
16. Thinking about how things should or shouldn't be	1	2	3	4	5	6	7	8	9	10

Physiological

17. Experiencing pain or discomfort	1	2	3	4	5	6	7	8	9	10

Nutrition

Physiological (continued)	Very Unlikely								Very Likely	
18. Experiencing trembling, headache, or lightheadedness associated with no eating or too much caffeine	1	2	3	4	5	6	7	8	9	10
19. Experiencing fatigue or feeling overtired	1	2	3	4	5	6	7	8	9	10
20. Experiencing hunger pangs or urges to eat, even though I've eaten recently	1	2	3	4	5	6	7	8	9	10

Scoring

Total your scores for each area and enter them below. Then rank the scores by marking the highest score "1," next highest score "2," and so on. Focus on the highest-ranked areas first, but any score above 24 is high and indicates that you need to work on that area.

Area	Total Score	Rank Score
Social (Items 1–4)	_____	_____
Emotional (Items 5–8)	_____	_____
Situational (Items 9–12)	_____	_____
Thinking (Items 13–16)	_____	_____
Physiological (Items 17–20)	_____	_____

Lowering a High Score

Social Try reducing your susceptibility to the influence of others by communicating more assertively and rethinking your beliefs about obligations you feel you must fulfill.

Emotional Develop stress-management skills and practice positive self-talk to cope with emotions in ways that don't involve food.

Situational Work on controlling your environment and having a plan for handling external cues.

Thinking Change your thinking—be less self-critical and more flexible—to recognize rationalizations and excuses about eating behavior.

Physiological Look at the way you eat, what you eat, and medications to find ways these factors may be affecting your eating behavior.

Source: What Triggers Your Eating? Adapted from Nash, J. D. 1997. *The New Maximize Your Body Potential.* Palo Alto, Calif: Bull Publishing. Reprinted with permission from Bull Publishing Company.

POSTPROGRAM NUTRITION LOGS

Now that you have analyzed your diet and targeted some changes described in your Behavior Change Contract, you are ready to put your plan into action. Fill out this second nutrition log, again keeping a record of everything you eat for 3 consecutive days. Remember to record all foods and break down each food item into its component parts, listing them separately. Enter the portion sizes you consume in the correct food group column. For example, a turkey sandwich might be listed as follows: whole-wheat bread, 2 oz-equiv of whole grains; turkey, 2 oz-equiv of meat/beans; tomato, $1/3$ cup vegetables; romaine lettuce, $1/4$ cup vegetables; 1 tablespoon mayonnaise dressing, 1 teaspoon oils. Refer to Appendixes B and C in your text and the MyPyramid.gov Web site for additional guidelines. At the bottom of the chart, keep count of the number of servings of whole grains and the number of vegetable subgroups you consume daily (whole grains and vegetable subgroups are described on pp. 54–55).

Postprogram Nutrition Log

DAY 1

Food	Grains (oz-eq)	Vegetables (cups)	Fruit (cups)	Milk (cups)	Meat/beans (oz-eq)	Oils (tsp)	Solid fats (g)	Added sugars (g/tsp)
Daily total								

Number of servings of whole grains: ____
Number of vegetable subgroups consumed: ____

Postprogram Nutrition Log

DAY 2

Food	Grains (oz-eq)	Vegetables (cups)	Fruit (cups)	Milk (cups)	Meat/beans (oz-eq)	Oils (tsp)	Solid fats (g)	Added sugars (g/tsp)
Daily total								

Number of servings of whole grains: _____
Number of vegetable subgroups consumed: _____

Nutrition

Postprogram Nutrition Log

DAY 3

Food	Grains (oz-eq)	Vegetables (cups)	Fruit (cups)	Milk (cups)	Meat/beans (oz-eq)	Oils (tsp)	Solid fats (g)	Added sugars (g/tsp)
Daily total								

Number of servings of whole grains: ____
Number of vegetable subgroups consumed: ____

ASSESSING IMPROVEMENT IN YOUR DAILY DIET

Fill in your recommended MyPyramid intakes from p. 51 and then the daily totals from your 3 days of postprogram food logs. Average your daily totals and compare them to the MyPyramid recommendations and to your preprogram average (from p. 65).

Group	Day 1	Day 2	Day 3	Average of 3 days (postprogram)	Average of 3 days (preprogram)	MyPyramid recommended totals
Grains (oz-eq)						
Whole grains (oz-eq)						
Vegetables (cups)						
# of subgroups						
Fruit (cups)						
Milk (cups)						
Meat/beans (oz-eq)						
Oils (tsp)						
Solid fats (g)						
Added sugars (g/tsp)						

In comparing the results of my postprogram log to the results of my preprogram log, I found that

_____

_____

_____

_____

Nutrition

Completing a Behavior Change Contract and following its steps helped me to

_____

_____

_____

_____

_____

Areas of improvement that I will focus on in the future are

_____

_____

_____

_____

_____

_____

_____

You can use the additional logs that follow (pp. 79–85) to track your diet in the future; for tips on weight management, go to p. 86.

Nutrition

Nutrition Log

Date _____

Food	Grains (oz-eq)	Vegetables (cups)	Fruit (cups)	Milk (cups)	Meat/beans (oz-eq)	Oils (tsp)	Solid fats (g)	Added sugars (g/tsp)
Daily total								

Number of servings of whole grains: ____
Number of vegetable subgroups consumed: ____

Nutrition Log

Date _____

Food	Grains (oz-eq)	Vegetables (cups)	Fruit (cups)	Milk (cups)	Meat/beans (oz-eq)	Oils (tsp)	Solid fats (g)	Added sugars (g/tsp)
Daily total								

Number of servings of whole grains: ____
Number of vegetable subgroups consumed: ____

Nutrition Log

Date _____

Food	Grains (oz-eq)	Vegetables (cups)	Fruit (cups)	Milk (cups)	Meat/beans (oz-eq)	Oils (tsp)	Solid fats (g)	Added sugars (g/tsp)
Daily total								

Number of servings of whole grains: _____
Number of vegetable subgroups consumed: _____

Nutrition Log

Date _____

Food	Grains (oz-eq)	Vegetables (cups)	Fruit (cups)	Milk (cups)	Meat/beans (oz-eq)	Oils (tsp)	Solid fats (g)	Added sugars (g/tsp)
Daily total								

Number of servings of whole grains: ____
Number of vegetable subgroups consumed: ____

Nutrition Log

Date _____

Food	Grains (oz-eq)	Vegetables (cups)	Fruit (cups)	Milk (cups)	Meat/beans (oz-eq)	Oils (tsp)	Solid fats (g)	Added sugars (g/tsp)
Daily total								

Number of servings of whole grains: _____
Number of vegetable subgroups consumed: _____

Nutrition Log

Date _____

Food	Grains (oz-eq)	Vegetables (cups)	Fruit (cups)	Milk (cups)	Meat/beans (oz-eq)	Oils (tsp)	Solid fats (g)	Added sugars (g/tsp)
Daily total								

Number of servings of whole grains: ____
Number of vegetable subgroups consumed: ____

Nutrition Log

Date _____

Food	Grains (oz-eq)	Vegetables (cups)	Fruit (cups)	Milk (cups)	Meat/beans (oz-eq)	Oils (tsp)	Solid fats (g)	Added sugars (g/tsp)
Daily total								

Number of servings of whole grains: ____
Number of vegetable subgroups consumed: ____

WEIGHT MANAGEMENT

CREATING A WEIGHT MANAGEMENT PROGRAM

Completing the preprogram and postprogram nutrition logs will help you monitor and improve your daily diet. If you decide that your weight or percent body fat is above or below the amount that is appropriate for your size, gender, and age, the information you have gathered with your nutrition logs will be an important part of a weight management program. This section outlines the general steps in a weight management program; in the next section you'll track activity and food choices to identify ways to create a negative energy balance and lose weight.

Follow these steps to develop your weight management program and put it into action:

1. Assess Your Motivation and Commitment

Make sure you are motivated and committed to your plan for weight management before you begin. It is important to understand why you want to change your weight or body composition. You will generally be more successful if your reasons are self-focused, such as wanting to feel good about yourself, rather than connected to others' perceptions of you.

When you understand your reasons for wanting to manage your weight, list them below. Post your list in a prominent place as a reminder.

1. _____

2. _____

3. _____

4. _____

2. Set Goals

After you have chosen a reasonable long-term weight or body-fat percentage goal, break your progress into a series of short-term goals. You can include a small, non-food-related reward like a new CD or a night at the movies for successfully reaching each goal.

Goal	Reward
1. _____	_____
2. _____	_____
3. _____	_____
4. _____	_____

3. Assess Your Current Energy Balance

When your weight is stable, you are burning approximately the same number of calories that you are taking in. In order to lose weight, you must consume fewer calories, burn more calories through physical activity, or both. This will create a negative energy balance that will lead to gradual, moderate weight loss. Strategies for creating a negative energy balance are discussed on page 89 of this journal.

4. Increase Your Level of Physical Activity

You can increase your energy output simply by increasing your routine physical activity, such as walking or taking the stairs. You will increase your energy output even more if you adopt a program of regular exercise like the one described in the first section of this journal.

5. Evaluate Your Diet and Eating Habits

Take another look at the nutrition logs you completed. Are there some high-calorie, low-nutrient foods that stand out? If your increase in physical activity does not result in a negative energy balance that produces weight loss, you may want to make small cuts in your calorie intake by reducing your consumption of these foods.

Weight Management

6. Track Your Physical Activity and Diet

Use the weight management logs to record your daily physical activities and dietary choices. These logs will help you uncover potential calorie savings that will create a negative calorie balance and help you lose weight.

For People Who Want to Gain Weight

If the goal of your weight management program is to increase your weight, you'll need to create a positive energy balance by taking in more calories than you use. The basis of a successful and healthy program for weight gain is a combination of strength training and a high-calorie diet. Strength training will help you add weight as muscle rather than as fat. To increase your calorie consumption, eat more high-carbohydrate foods, including grains, vegetables, and fruits. (Fatty, high-calorie foods may seem like a logical choice for weight gain, but a diet high in fat carries health risks, and your body is likely to convert dietary fat into body fat rather than into muscle.) Avoid skipping meals, add two or three snacks to your daily diet, and consider adding a dietary supplement high in carbohydrates, protein, vitamins, and minerals. As with weight loss, a gradual program of weight gain is the best strategy.

CREATING A NEGATIVE ENERGY BALANCE

A reasonable weight-loss goal is ½–1 pound per week. Depending on your individual characteristics, you will need to create a negative energy balance of between 1750 and 3500 calories a week, or 250–500 calories a day. While this may seem daunting, you already make choices every day that affect your energy balance significantly. Making a few decisions each day with your energy balance in mind can add up to a successful weight management program.

First, review the sample weight management log on the next page that shows the daily activities of Elizabeth, a hypothetical 21-year-old student weighing 130 pounds. As she goes through her day, she has many opportunities to make choices that will affect her energy balance. In the real world, you will be more likely to make one or two choices each day that decrease the number of calories you take in or increase the number of calories you expend. The key is to be aware of your opportunities to affect your energy balance and to make healthy choices as often as possible without making yourself feel deprived.

After you have reviewed this example, record and assess your own daily choices using the blank weight management logs that follow. Fill in your activities and your meals and snacks, and then think about alternatives you could have chosen. What would the potential calorie savings have been if you had made these choices? To calculate the calories you expended in physical activity, consult the table of common sports and fitness activities on page 90 of this journal, information in your text, and materials on energy balance in the report from the Surgeon General on physical activity and the Surgeon General's Call to Action on obesity (available online at www.surgeongeneral.gov). To calculate calories saved by making a healthier food choice, use information in your text, the fast food data available at the back of this journal, and the USDA online nutrient database (www.nal.usda.gov/fnic/foodcomp/search).

Weight Management

CALORIE COSTS FOR COMMON SPORTS AND FITNESS ACTIVITIES

When you change your energy balance by participating in an activity that expends calories, how do you calculate how many calories you have actually spent? Calorie costs are given here for 10 common activities; use these as benchmarks for calculating the calorie costs of other activities.

Multiply the number in the appropriate column (moderate or vigorous) by your body weight and then by the number of minutes you exercise. (If you participate in your activity at a level between moderate and vigorous, use a number between the two values.) For example, if you weigh 150 pounds and play tennis vigorously for 45 minutes, multiply .071 (value) by 150 (weight) and then by 45 (time) for a result of 479 calories expended.

	Approximate Calorie Cost	
Activity	*Moderate*	*Vigorous*
Aerobic dance	.046	.062
Basketball, half court	.045	.071
Bicycling	.049	.071
Hiking	.051	.073
Jogging and running	.060	.104
Racquetball, skilled, singles	.049	.078
Skating, ice, roller, and in-line	.049	.095
Swimming	.032	.088
Tennis, skilled, singles	—	.071
Walking	.029	.048

Sample Daily Weight Management Log

Activity/Meal or Snack	Healthier Choice (describe)	Approximate Calorie Savings
Friday morning, Elizabeth eats breakfast: a croissant and a cup of coffee with cream.	Friday morning, Elizabeth eats breakfast: a bowl of whole-grain cereal, a glass of orange juice, and a cup of coffee. She uses most of a glass of skim milk for her cereal and puts the rest in her coffee.	81
Elizabeth drives to campus.	Elizabeth walks 15 minutes to campus.	57
After class, Elizabeth visits her friend's dorm, where they watch the noon soap opera for an hour.	After class, Elizabeth meets her friend for a 25-minute jog.	195
For lunch, Elizabeth eats 2 slices of leftover pepperoni pizza and drinks a soda.	After their jog, they have lunch at the dorm; each has a turkey sandwich, an apple, and iced tea.	231
Elizabeth goes to her afternoon class. She wants a snack, so she buys a candy bar from the vending machine.	Elizabeth goes to her afternoon class. She wants a snack, so she buys a nonfat yogurt with fruit in the student union.	142
Elizabeth drives home.	Elizabeth walks 15 minutes home.	57
Elizabeth studies until her roommates get home.	Elizabeth studies until her roommates get home.	—
Elizabeth and her roommates decide to stop for fast food on the way to the movies. Elizabeth orders a cheeseburger, large french fries, and a small chocolate shake.	Elizabeth and her roommates decide to stop for fast food on the way to the movies. Elizabeth orders a hamburger, a green salad with carrots and fat-free dressing, and a small chocolate shake.	389
At the movies, Elizabeth shares a bag of buttered popcorn with her friend.	At the movies, Elizabeth shares a bag of air-popped popcorn with her friend.	64

Weight Management

Daily Weight Management Log

Activity/Meal or Snack	Healthier Choice (describe)	Approximate Calorie Savings

Daily Weight Management Log

Activity/Meal or Snack	Healthier Choice (describe)	Approximate Calorie Savings

Weight Management

Daily Weight Management Log

Activity/Meal or Snack	Healthier Choice (describe)	Approximate Calorie Savings

Daily Weight Management Log

Activity/Meal or Snack	Healthier Choice (describe)	Approximate Calorie Savings

Weight Management

Daily Weight Management Log

Activity/Meal or Snack	Healthier Choice (describe)	Approximate Calorie Savings

Weight Management

Daily Weight Management Log

Activity/Meal or Snack	Healthier Choice (describe)	Approximate Calorie Savings

Daily Weight Management Log

Activity/Meal or Snack	Healthier Choice (describe)	Approximate Calorie Savings

Daily Weight Management Log

Activity/Meal or Snack	Healthier Choice (describe)	Approximate Calorie Savings

Weight Management

Daily Weight Management Log

Activity/Meal or Snack	Healthier Choice (describe)	Approximate Calorie Savings

APPENDIX Nutritional Content of Popular Items from Fast-Food Restaurants

Arby's

	Serving size (g)	Calories	Protein (g)	Total fat (g)	Saturated fat (g)	Total carbohydrate (g)	Sugars (g)	Fiber (g)	Cholesterol (mg)	Sodium (mg)	Vitamin A	Vitamin C	Calcium	Iron	% Calories from fat
											% Daily Value				
Regular roast beef	154	320	21	13	6	34	5	2	45	950	0	0	6	20	34
Super roast beef	241	440	22	19	7	48	11	3	45	1130	2	2	8	25	39
Junior roast beef	125	270	16	9	4	34	5	2	30	740	0	0	6	15	33
Market Fresh® Ultimate BLT	293	780	23	46	9	75	18	6	50	1570	15	30	15	25	53
Market Fresh® Roast Turkey & Swiss	357	720	45	27	6	74	16	5	90	1790	8	4	35	30	35
Market Fresh® Low Carbys™ Southwest chicken wrap	259	550	35	30	9	45	1	30	75	1690	10	10	40	10	49
Chicken breast fillet	204	490	25	24	4	46	7	2	55	1220	2	2	8	15	44
Martha's Vineyard™ salad (w/o dressing)	291	250	26	8	4.5	23	23	4	60	490	60	40	20	10	28
Raspberry vinaigrette	57	172	0	12	1.5	16	14	0	0	344	0	4	0	0	63
Santa Fe™ salad (w/o dressing)	328	520	27	29	9	40	6	5	60	1120	130	45	25	20	50
Curly fries (medium)	128	410	5	22	3	47	N/A	5	0	950	8	10	6	10	49
Jalapeno Bites®, regular (5)	110	310	5	19	7	29	3	2	30	530	15	0	4	6	55
Chocolate shake, regular	397	510	13	13	0	83	81	0	35	360	8	10	50	2	23

SOURCE: Arby's © 2005, Arby's, Inc. (http://www.arbysrestaurant.com). Used with permission of Arby's, Inc.

Burger King

	Serving size (g)	Calories	Protein (g)	Total fat (g)	Saturated fat (g)	Trans fat (g)	Total Carbohydrate (g)	Sugars (g)	Fiber (g)	Cholesterol (mg)	Sodium (mg)	Vitamin A	Vitamin C	Calcium	Iron	% calories from fat
												% Daily Value				
Whopper®	291	700	31	42	13	1	52	8	4	85	1020	20	15	10	30	54
Whopper® w/o mayonnaise	270	540	30	24	10	1	52	8	4	75	900	10	15	10	30	40
Double Whopper® w/cheese	399	1060	56	69	27	2.5	53	9	4	185	1540	25	15	30	45	59
Whopper Jr.®	158	390	17	22	7	0.5	31	5	2	45	550	10	6	8	15	51
BK Veggie® Burger*	215	420	23	16	3	0	46	7	7	10	1090	20	10	10	20	34
Original Chicken Sandwich	204	560	25	28	6	2	52	5	3	60	1270	8	0	6	15	45
Chicken Tenders® (8 pieces)	123	340	22	19	5	3.5	20	0	<1	50	840	2	0	2	4	50
French fries (medium, salted)	117	360	4	18	5	4.5	46	<1	4	0	640	0	15	2	4	45
Onion rings (medium)	91	320	4	16	4	3.5	40	5	3	0	460	0	0	10	0	45
Tendergrill™ Chicken Caesar Salad w/o dressing	299	220	31	7	3	0	7	1	2	60	710	80	40	20	10	29
Ken's ranch dressing (2 oz)	57	190	1	20	3	0	2	1	0	20	550	0	0	2	0	95
Croissan'wich® w/ bacon, egg & cheese	122	340	15	20	7	2	26	5	<1	155	890	8	15	15	10	53
Hershey®'s sundae pie	79	300	3	18	10	1.5	31	23	1	10	190	2	0	4	6	54
Chocolate shake (medium)	447	690	11	20	12	0	114	110	2	75	560	15	6	45	10	26

SOURCE: BURGER KING® nutritional information used with permission from Burger King Brands, Inc. (http://www.burgerking.com)

Domino's Pizza
(1 of 8 equal slices)

	Serving size (g)	Calories	Protein (g)	Total fat (g)	Saturated fat (g)	Total carbohydrate (g)	Sugars (g)	Fiber (g)	Cholesterol (mg)	Sodium (mg)	Vitamin A	Vitamin C	Calcium	Iron	% calories from fat
											% Daily Value				
14-inch lg. hand tossed cheese	110	256	10	8	3	38	3	2	12	535.5	8	0	12	11	26
14-inch lg. thin crust cheese	68	188	7	10	3.5	19	2	1	13	408.5	8	4	12	4	40
14-inch lg. deep dish cheese	128	336	13	15	5	41	4	2	16	782	10	0	16	15	40
12-inch med. hand tossed cheese	79	186	7	5.5	2	28	2	1	9	385	6	0	9	8	26
12-inch med. thin crust cheese	49	137	5	7	2.5	14	2	1	10	292.5	6	3	9	3	40
12-inch med. deep dish cheese	90	238	9	11	3.5	28	3	2	11	555.5	7	0	11	11	41
14-inch lg. hand tossed pepperoni & sausage	130	350	14	16	6	39	3	2	31	863	9	0	14	13	41
14-inch lg. hand tossed ham & pineapple	130	275	12	8.5	3.5	40	5	2	17	653	8	2	12	12	28
14-inch lg. hand tossed ExtravaganZZa Feast®	165	388	17	18.5	7.5	40	3	3	37	1014	12	2	19	15	43
14-inch lg. hand tossed Hawaiian Feast®	141	309	14	11	4.5	41	5	2	23	765	11	2	18	13	32
14-inch lg. thin crust Vegi Feast®	97	231	10	13.5	5	21	3	2	19	550.5	11	5	18	6	53
14-inch lg. deep dish MeatZZa Feast®	167	458	19	25	9.5	42	4	3	40	1230	13	1	22	18	49
Barbecue buffalo wings (1 piece)	25	50	6	2.5	0.5	2	1	<1	26	175.5	1	0	1	2	36
Buffalo Chicken Kickers™ (1 piece)	24	47	4	2	0.5	3	0	0	9	162.5	0	0	0	0	38
Blue cheese sauce	43	223	1	23.5	4	2	2	0	20	417	1	0	2	0	93
Breadsticks (1 stick)	30	115	2	6.3	1.1	12	1	0	0	122.1	4	0	0	4	31
Cinna Stix® (1 stick)	30	123	2	6.1	1.1	15	3	1	0	111	4	0	0	4	45

KFC

	Serving size (g)	Calories	Protein (g)	Total fat (g)	Saturated fat (g)	Trans fat (g)	Total carbohydrate (g)	Sugars (g)	Fiber (g)	Cholesterol (mg)	Sodium (mg)	Vitamin A (% Daily Value)	Vitamin C (% Daily Value)	Calcium (% Daily Value)	Iron (% Daily Value)	% Calories from fat
Original Recipe® breast	161	380	40	19	6	2.5	11	0	0	145	1150	0	0	0	6	45
Original Recipe® thigh	126	360	22	25	7	1.5	12	0	0	165	1060	0	0	0	6	63
Extra Crispy™ breast	162	460	34	28	8	4.5	19	0	0	135	1230	0	0	0	8	55
Extra Crispy™ thigh	114	370	21	26	7	3	12	0	0	120	710	0	0	0	6	63
Tender Roast® sandwich w/ sauce	196	390	31	19	4	0.5	24	0	1	70	810	0	4	4	10	44
Tender Roast® sandwich w/o sauce	177	260	31	5	1.5	0.5	23	0	1	65	690	0	4	4	10	17
Tender Roast® Filet Meal	321	360	33	7	2	0.5	41	4	4	85	2010	20	6	6	15	18
Hot Wings™ (6 pieces)	134	450	24	29	6	4	23	1	1	145	1120	6	8	8	10	58
Popcorn chicken (large)	170	560	36	31	7	7	34	0	1	90	1790	4	4	0	15	50
Chicken pot pie	423	770	33	40	15	14	70	2	5	115	1680	200	0	0	20	47
Roasted Caesar Salad w/o dressing and croutons	301	220	29	9	4.5	0.5	6	4	3	75	850	45	35	25	10	37
KFC® creamy parmesan Caesar dressing	57	260	2	26	5	0.25	5	3	0	15	530	0	2	2	0	90
Corn on the cob (5.5 in.)	162	150	5	3	1	0	26	10	7	0	10	0	6	6	6	18
Mashed potatoes w/ gravy	136	120	2	4.5	1	0.5	18	<1	1	0	380	10	0	2	2	34
Baked beans	136	230	8	1	1	0.25	46	22	7	0	720	4	15	30	30	4
Cole slaw	130	190	1	11	2	0.25	22	13	3	5	300	40	4	0	0	52
Biscuit (1)	57	190	2	10	2	3.5	23	1	0	1.5	580	0	0	0	4	47
Potato salad	128	180	2	9	1.5	0.25	22	5	1	5	470	10	0	0	2	45

SOURCE: KFC Corporation, 2005. Nutritional information provided by KFC Corporation from its website www.kfc.com as of September 2005 and subject to the conditions listed therein. KFC and related marks are registered trademarks of KFC Corporation. Reproduced with permission from Kentucky Fried Chicken Corporation.

McDonald's

	Serving size (g)	Calories	Protein (g)	Total fat (g)	Saturated fat (g)	Trans fat (g)	Total carbohydrate (g)	Sugars (g)	Fiber (g)	Cholesterol (mg)	Sodium (mg)	Vitamin A	Vitamin C	Calcium	Iron	% calories from fat
												(% Daily Value)				
Hamburger	105	260	13	9	3.5	0.5	33	7	1	30	530	2	2	15	15	31
Quarter Pounder®	171	420	13	9	3.5	0.5	33	7	1	30	530	2	2	15	15	46
Quarter Pounder® w/ cheese	199	510	29	25	12	1.5	43	9	3	95	1150	10	2	30	25	43
Big Mac®	219	560	25	30	10	1.5	47	8	3	80	1010	8	2	25	25	48
Big N' Tasty®	232	470	24	23	8	1.5	41	9	3	80	790	8	8	15	25	50
Filet-O-Fish®	141	400	14	18	4	1	42	8	1	40	640	2	0	15	10	40
McChicken®	147	370	15	16	3.5	1	41	5	1	50	810	2	2	15	15	48
Medium French Fries	114	350	4	16	3	4	47	0	5	0	220	0	10	2	6	43
Chicken McNuggets® (6 pieces)	96	250	15	15	3	1.5	15	0	0	35	670	2	2	2	4	52
Chicken Select® Premium Breast Strips	221	630	39	33	6	4.5	46	0	0	90	1550	0	6	4	8	48
Tangy Honey Mustard Sauce	43	70	1	2	0	0	13	9	1	0	160	0	0	0	1	29
Bacon Ranch Salad w/ Grilled Chicken (w/o dressing)	320	260	33	9	4	0	12	5	3	90	1000	120	15	15	10	33
Caesar Salad w/Crispy Chicken (w/o dressing)	313	300	25	13	4	1.5	22	4	3	55	1020	120	20	20	10	40
California Cobb Salad (w/o chicken and dressing)	2374	160	11	9	4	0	9	5	4	85	410	120	15	15	8	53
Newman's Own® Ranch Dressing (2 oz)	59	170	1	15	2.5	0	9	4	0	20	530	0	4	4	0	76
Egg McMuffin®	138	290	17	11	4.5	0	30	2	2	235	850	10	2	30	14	34
Sausage Biscuit w/ Egg	162	500	18	32	10	5	36	2	1	250	1080	6	0	8	20	58
Hotcakes (2 pats margarine & syrup)	221	600	9	17	4	4	102	45	2	20	620	8	0	15	15	27
Fruit 'n Yogurt Parfait	149	160	4	2	1	0	31	21	<1	5	85	0	15	15	4	13
Chocolate Triple Thick® Shake (16 oz)	444	580	13	14	8	1	102	84	<1	50	250	20	45	45	10	21

SOURCE: McDonald's Corporation, 2005 (http://www.mcdonalds.com). Used with permission from McDonald's Corporation.

Subway

Based on standard formulas with
6-inch subs on Italian or wheat bread

	Serving size (g)	Calories	Protein (g)	Total fat (g)	Saturated fat (g)	Trans fat (g)	Total carbohydrate (g)	Sugars (g)	Fiber (g)	Cholesterol (mg)	Sodium (mg)	Vitamin A	Vitamin C	Calcium	Iron	% calories from fat
Italian BMT®	242	450	23	21	8	0	47	8	4	55	1790	8	30	15	25	42
Meatball Marinara	377	560	24	24	11	1	63	13	7	45	1610	10	50	20	40	39
Subway® Seafood Sensation	250	450	16	22	6	0.5	51	8	5	25	1150	8	30	15	25	44
Cheese Steak	250	360	24	10	4.5	0	47	9	5	35	1100	8	30	15	45	25
Subway® Melt	254	380	25	12	5	0	48	8	4	45	1610	8	30	10	25	28
Tuna	250	530	22	31	7	0.5	45	7	4	45	1030	8	30	10	30	53
Sweet Onion Chicken Teriyaki	281	370	26	5	1.5	0	59	19	4	50	1220	6	40	8	25	12
Roast Beef	223	290	19	5	2	0	45	8	4	15	920	4	30	6	30	16
Turkey Breast	224	280	18	4.5	1.5	0	46	7	4	20	1020	4	30	4	25	14
Veggie Delite®	167	230	9	3	1	0	44	7	4	0	520	4	30	6	25	12
Turkey Breast Deli Style	152	210	13	3.5	1.5	0	36	4	3	15	730	4	15	6	25	15
Chicken & Bacon Ranch Wrap (w/ cheese)	256	440	41	27	10	0.5	18	1	9	90	1670	10	15	30	15	55
Turkey Breast Wrap	183	190	24	6	1	0	18	2	9	20	1290	4	10	10	15	28
Grilled Chicken & Baby Spinach Salad (w/o dressing)	300	140	20	3	1	0	11	4	4	50	450	200	80	10	20	19
Tuna (w/ cheese) Salad (w/o dressing)	404	360	16	29	6	0.5	12	5	4	45	600	70	50	15	15	73
New England Clam Chowder	240	110	5	3.5	0.5	0	16	1	1	10	990	2	2	10	4	29
Chili Con Carne	240	240	15	10	5	0	23	14	8	15	860	15	0	6	10	38
Sunrise Refresher (small)	341	120	1	0	0	0	29	28	1	0	20	4	210	2	0	0
Western Breakfast Sandwich w/ Cheese	211	400	27	14	7	0	46	6	4	40	1210	6	20	25	25	32
Chocolate Chip Cookie	45	210	2	10	4	1	30	18	1	15	160	4	0	0	6	43

Taco Bell

	Serving size (g)	Calories	Protein (g)	Total fat (g)	Saturated fat (g)	Trans fat (g)	Total Carbohydrate (g)	Sugars (g)	Fiber (g)	Cholesterol (mg)	Sodium (mg)	Vitamin A (% DV)	Vitamin C (% DV)	Calcium (% DV)	Iron (% DV)	% Calories from fat
Taco	92	150	7	7	2.5	0.5	14	1	2	20	360	4	4	2	6	53
Taco Supreme®	113	220	9	14	7	1	14	2	1	35	360	8	6	8	6	57
Soft taco, beef	99	210	10	10	4	1	21	2	1	25	620	4	0	10	8	43
Gordita Supreme®, steak	153	290	16	13	5	0.5	28	7	2	35	520	6	6	10	15	37
Gordita Baja®, chicken	153	320	17	15	5	0	29	7	2	40	690	6	6	10	10	42
Gordita Baja®, chicken, "Fresco Style"	153	230	15	6	1	0	29	7	2	25	570	10	10	6	10	23
Chalupa Supreme, beef	153	390	14	24	10	3	31	4	1	35	600	6	6	15	8	55
Chalupa Supreme, chicken	153	370	17	20	8	3	30	4	1	45	530	8	8	10	6	49
Bean burrito	198	370	14	10	3.5	2	55	4	8	10	1200	8	8	20	15	24
Burrito Supreme®, chicken	248	410	21	14	6	2	50	5	5	45	1270	15	15	20	15	31
Grilled stuffed burrito, beef	325	720	27	33	11	3.5	79	6	7	55	2090	15	6	35	25	41
Tostada	170	250	11	10	4	1.5	29	2	7	15	710	10	8	15	8	36
Zesty Chicken Border Bowl™ w/dressing	418	730	23	42	9	4	65	5	12	45	1640	20	15	15	20	52
Fiesta taco salad	548	870	31	47	16	9	80	10	12	65	1780	20	40	35	35	49
Steak quesadilla	184	540	26	31	14	2	40	4	3	70	1370	15	2	50	15	52
Nachos Supreme	195	450	13	26	9	5	42	3	5	35	810	8	8	10	10	58
Nachos BellGrande®	308	780	20	43	13	10	80	5	11	35	1300	8	8	20	15	50
Pintos 'n cheese	128	180	10	7	3.5	1	20	1	6	15	700	6	6	15	6	35
Mexican rice	131	210	6	10	4	1.5	23	<1	3	15	740	8	8	10	10	43

SOURCE: Taco Bell Corporation, 2005 (http://www.tacobell.com). Reproduced courtesy of Taco Bell Corporation.

Wendy's

	Serving size (g)	Calories	Protein (g)	Total fat (g)	Saturated fat (g)	Trans fat (g)	Total Carbohydrate (g)	Sugars (g)	Fiber (g)	Cholesterol (mg)	Sodium (mg)	Vitamin A	Vitamin C	Calcium	Iron	% Calories from fat
												% Daily Value				
Classic Single® w/ everything	218	430	25	20	7	1	37	8	2	65	890	8	10	4	25	42
Big Bacon Classic®	282	580	35	29	12	1.5	46	11	3	95	1390	20	20	15	30	45
Jr. Hamburger	117	280	15	9	3.5	0.5	34	7	1	30	600	2	2	2	20	30
Jr. Bacon Cheeseburger	165	380	20	18	7	0.5	34	6	2	55	810	10	10	10	20	45
Ultimate Chicken Grill Sandwich	225	360	31	7	1.5	0	44	10	2	75	1090	15	30	4	15	18
Spicy Chicken Fillet Sandwich	225	510	29	19	3.5	1.5	57	8	2	55	1480	15	10	4	20	34
Homestyle Chicken Fillet Sandwich	230	540	29	22	4	1.5	57	8	2	55	1320	15	15	4	20	37
Homestyle Chicken Strips (3)	159	410	28	18	3.5	3	33	0	0	60	1470	0	0	2	6	40
Caesar Side Salad (no toppings or dressing)	99	70	6	4.5	2	0	3	1	2	15	150	100	10	10	0	58
Mandarin Chicken® Salad (no toppings or dressing)	348	170	23	2	0.5	0	18	13	3	60	480	70	50	6	10	11
Taco Supremo salad (no toppings or dressing)	494	380	27	17	9	0.5	31	9	9	65	1000	70	35	35	20	40
Creamy ranch dressing	64	230	1	23	4	0.5	5	3	0	15	580	0	4	4	2	90
Reduced fat creamy ranch dressing	64	100	1	8	1.5	0	6	3	1	15	550	0	4	4	2	72
Biggie® fries	159	490	5	24	4	6	65	0	6	0	480	4	10	2	8	39
Broccoli & Cheese Baked Potato	397	340	10	3.5	1	0	69	6	9	10	430	10	110	20	20	9
Fresh Fruit Bowl	297	130	2	0	0	0	33	28	3	0	35	100	150	4	6	0
Chili, small, plain	227	220	17	6	2.5	0	23	6	5	35	780	4	4	8	15	23
Crispy Chicken Nuggets™ (5)	75	220	10	14	3	1.5	13	1	0	35	490	0	0	0	2	57
Barbecue sauce (1 packet)	28	40	1	0	0	0	11	5	0	0	160	0	0	0	4	0
Frosty,™ medium	298	430	10	11	7	0	74	55	0	45	200	20	40	20	20	23

SOURCE: Wendy's International, Inc.., 2005 (http://www.wendys.com). Reproduced with permission from Wendy's International, Inc. The information contained in Wendy's International Information is effective as of August 2005. Wendy's International, Inc., its subsidiaries, affiliates, franchises, and employees do not assume responsibility for a particular sensitivity or allergy (including peanuts, nuts or other allergies) to any food product provided in our restaurants. We encourage anyone with food sensitivities, allergies, or special dietary needs to check on a regular basis with Wendy's Consumer Relations Department to obtain the most up-to-date information.